Nathacha Barroso Rosa

Occupational Therapy in the prevention of Postpartum Depression

Nathacha Barroso Rosa

Occupational Therapy in the prevention of Postpartum Depression

Occupational therapy as a strategy for preventing post-natal depression in the prenatal period

ScienciaScripts

Imprint

Any brand names and product names mentioned in this book are subject to trademark, brand or patent protection and are trademarks or registered trademarks of their respective holders. The use of brand names, product names, common names, trade names, product descriptions etc. even without a particular marking in this work is in no way to be construed to mean that such names may be regarded as unrestricted in respect of trademark and brand protection legislation and could thus be used by anyone.

Cover image: www.ingimage.com

This book is a translation from the original published under ISBN 978-613-9-73055-1.

Publisher:
Sciencia Scripts
is a trademark of
Dodo Books Indian Ocean Ltd. and OmniScriptum S.R.L publishing group

120 High Road, East Finchley, London, N2 9ED, United Kingdom
Str. Armeneasca 28/1, office 1, Chisinau MD-2012, Republic of Moldova, Europe
Printed at: see last page
ISBN: 978-620-7-88835-1

DEDICATORY

I dedicate this book to my son Gael, the greatest love of my life!

ACKNOWLEDGEMENTS

The realisation of this work was only possible thanks to the direct and indirect collaboration of many people. I would like to express my gratitude to all of them and in particular: to God; to my parents Maria Das Graças and Carlos Alberto, who never spared any effort for my education; to my supervisor Prof Márcia Monteiro Garcia; to my friend Camille Santos Silva; to my family and friends for their understanding in times of absence.

SUMMARY

Summary

This paper presents research carried out at the Women's Health Integrated Coordination Centre in the municipality of Carmo, Rio de Janeiro. This programme is offered to puerperal women and shows why cases of post-natal depression have low reliability or are not always correctly treated. The paper also shows the results of a survey of women who have already experienced post-natal depression, their feelings, fears, anxieties and what they think about a programme of occupational therapeutic care from prenatal onwards. The structured results were obtained by applying a self-structured instrument adapted from the Edinburgh Depression Scale (EPDS) to women who had already been diagnosed with post-natal depression, in a universe of 120 women treated at the Women's Health Integrated Coordination Centre. Occupational therapy provides important resources for pregnant women who want to prevent post-natal depression, as well as for puerperal women who already have depression.

Keywords: Postpartum Depression. SUS. Occupational Therapy. Prenatal care.

CHAPTER 1

INTRODUCTION

According to Genesis, one of the greatest glories in a woman's life is motherhood. In ancient cultures, including Israel, the importance of women was centred on motherhood, from the virginal stage, the preparation for marriage, to the family stage, where the mother came to dominate other functions (Genesis 2:18).

Woman was considered a secondary being, made for man and destined for his happiness. The Yahweh account of creation shows that she was created after man, taken from his flesh, as a part of man destined to help him. Woman's punishment for sin is represented by her dependence on man and the pain of childbirth (GENESIS, 13,16).

Contemporary society is completely competitive and capitalist. Where women are concerned, social demands are even greater. Today, women work, study hard and are extremely dedicated to their goals. As a result, she gets pregnant later, when she's already full of problems and information. The professional, personal, social and physical demands imposed by modern society can trigger psychiatric conditions, including post-natal depression, according to Joel Rennó Júnior, PhD in psychiatry from USP's Faculty of Medicine (Brazilian Association of Psychiatry, accessed in November 2008).

According to CURY (2007), if Mary, the mother of Jesus Christ, had not protected herself emotionally, she would have developed psychological disorders. Young Mary's responsibility was great. Until she learnt to use her intuition in raising her son, her thoughts must have troubled her: how to raise this boy? What to do when he cries? Will he react like an ordinary child? Will I be able to raise my voice when I need to? And if he doesn't obey me, what should I do? If I fail, could I jeopardise the formation of his personality and, consequently, God's plans? What if I don't succeed?

Some mothers develop post-natal depression not just because of metabolic deficiencies and hormonal changes, but because, shackled by thoughts that reveal low self-esteem, they feel incapable of looking after their children, they believe that they are too fragile, that their body will never be the same again (CURY, 2007, p.94, 95).

Another point to be considered by Dr Rennó is that medicine is still unable to say precisely what causes a woman to develop post-natal depression. Studies show that the problem is the result of a great deal of interaction between biological, psychological and social factors (Associação Brasileira de Psiquiatria, accessed in November 2008).

Currently in Brazil, less than 25 per cent of affected puerperae have access to treatment, and only 50 per cent of cases of post-natal depression are diagnosed in the daily clinic (Revista de Psiquiatria do Rio Grande do Sul, 2007).

This paper presents research carried out at the Women's Health Integrated Coordination Centre in the municipality of Carmo, Rio de Janeiro. This programme is offered to postpartum women and shows why postpartum depression is unreliable or not always treated correctly.

The paper also shows the results of a survey of women who have experienced post-natal depression, their feelings, fears, anxieties and what they think about a programme of occupational therapy from prenatal onwards.

For these reasons, we were interested in formulating the following study questions: To detect the frequency of postpartum depression in puerperal women treated at the Integrated Coordination Centre for Women's, Children's and Adolescents' Health in the municipality of Carmo, RJ. To identify the demand for occupational therapy care for women during the prenatal period attended by the Integrated Coordination Centre for Women's, Children's and Adolescents' Health in the municipality of Carmo RJ. As for the intervention of Occupational Therapy in the care of women in the prenatal period and puerperal women with diagnosed postpartum depression.

By critically analysing the data collected through the research, we intend to show that Occupational Therapy makes an important contribution to the treatment of patients with post-natal depression.

CHAPTER 2

THEORETICAL BASIS

2.1 Post-natal depression

Postnatal depression results from a psychological and emotional moment of conflict and anguish that interferes with a woman's life. According to Kaplan and Sadock (2007), around 20 to 40 per cent of women report some emotional disturbance or cognitive dysfunction in the postnatal period. Many experience maternal sadness (baby blues), a normal state of sadness, dysphoria, frequent crying and dependence.

These feelings, which can last several days, have been attributed to rapid changes in hormone levels, the stress of childbirth and the awareness of the responsibility that motherhood brings. The condition is characterised by depressed mood, excessive anxiety and insomnia. It begins between 3 and 6 months after giving birth.

In rare cases (1 to 2 per 1000 births), postpartum depression is characterised by depressive feelings and suicidal ideation. In more serious situations, it can reach psychotic proportions, with hallucinations, delusions and thoughts of infanticide (KAPLAN & SADOCK, 2007, p.926).

"This is a severe and acute clinical condition that can begin in the first week after giving birth and last for up to two years," explains psychologist and psychotherapist Vera Iaconelli, who has a master's degree in psychology from the University of São Paulo (USP). (Brazilian Psychiatric Association, accessed November 2008).

Inability to care for and lack of interest in the baby are just two of the symptoms of PPD that harm not only the mother, but also the child.

It's worth pointing out that being overzealous with the baby can also be a sign of the disease. After giving birth, many mums are reluctant to admit to their family or even the child's father that they need help. This makes early diagnosis and, consequently, treatment of the problem more difficult.

Medicine is still unable to say precisely what causes a woman to develop post-natal depression. Studies show that the problem is the result of a great deal of interaction between biological, psychological and social factors. Women who have or have had some underlying pathology are more likely to suffer from it. Most women with postnatal depression have had a similar problem before, although of course this may be the first depressive manifestation in a woman's life. (Brazilian Psychiatric Association).

Some risk factors have been shown to correlate with PPD: women suffering from premenstrual tension (PMS), depressive symptoms during pregnancy, a history of affective disorders, first pregnancy, social deprivation, difficulties during pregnancy, complications during labour, being a single mother, marital conflicts.

In the postpartum period, depressive symptoms do not differ qualitatively from those that occur at other stages of life, and can be diagnosed and treated appropriately at the primary health care level. However, less than 25 per cent of affected puerperae have access to treatment, and only 50 per cent of cases of post-natal depression are diagnosed in the daily clinic (Revista de psiquiatria do Rio Grande do Sul, 2007).

2.2 Levels of depression and risk factors

The following tables are excerpts from a survey carried out by the ABP (Brazilian Psychiatry Association) in November 2008.

There are different clinical pictures of depression in the postpartum period.

TABLE 1: Minimum Level of Postnatal Psychic Disorder

BLUES (Mild disorder)
It affects around 70 *to* 85 per cent of women. It appears in the first few days after giving birth or up to 14 days afterwards. Irritability, anxiety, constant crying and mood instability are some of the symptoms that characterise this condition.
RISK FACTORS: Depressive symptoms during pregnancy, a history of depression (even mild) and so-called premenstrual dysphoric disorder, a more severe form of what is known as PMS (premenstrual tension).

Source: Brazilian Psychiatric Association, November 2008.

This mild disorder affects many women in the days following the birth of their baby. The mother may experience sudden mood swings, such as feeling very happy and then very sad. Maternal sadness doesn't always require medical treatment; it usually helps to join a support group or talk to other mums.

TABLE 2: Average Level of Postnatal Psychic Disorder

POSTPARTUM DEPRESSION (PPD)
It appears *from* the first to the fourth month after giving birth (approximately), with the duration of a depressive episode at any other stage of life. As depression is incapacitating, the mother is prevented

from carrying out everyday tasks, including those relating to the baby. In this case, the woman is depressed, shows a high degree of guilt, anxiety, fear of causing suffering to the baby and obsessive thoughts.

RISK FACTORS:

Depression already at the time of pregnancy, a significant history of depression - especially previous post-natal depression, in which the woman is already very depressed shortly before having the baby, marital problems, lack of social support and stressful events during pregnancy.

Source: Brazilian Psychiatric Association, November 2008.

Postnatal depression can occur for a few days to months after the birth of any baby, not just the first. When a woman's normal life is affected, it's a sure sign that she should seek help. If a woman doesn't get treatment for postnatal depression, the symptoms can get worse and last up to a year. Depression should be treated with medication and therapy.

TABLE 3: Maximum Level of Postpartum Psychic Disorder

POST-PARTUM PSYCHOSIS (severe disorder)

A rarer case, it affects around 0.1% *or* 0.2% of women. It usually appears in the first postpartum period, lasting for weeks or months. The woman in this condition may experience hallucinations, rapid mood swings (from euphoria to depression), mental confusion, may end up being very aggressive towards her child and may even contemplate the idea of facilitating the death or killing her own newborn child.

RISK FACTORS:

People with a family or personal history of bipolar mood disorder, a mental illness, and/or a previous episode of psychosis.

Postpartum psychosis is a very serious mental illness. It can appear quickly, usually within the first three months after giving birth. Women suffering from postnatal psychosis need immediate treatment and most often require drug treatment. Sometimes the woman is hospitalised because she is at risk of harming the baby and herself.

According to Angerami (2006), the puerperium, like pregnancy, is a very vulnerable period for crises, due to the profound intra- and interpersonal changes triggered by childbirth.

Maldonado (1988) considers the puerperium to be the "fourth trimester" of pregnancy, considering it to be a transitional period lasting approximately three months after giving birth, particularly accentuated in the first child. In this period, the woman becomes especially sensitive, often confused, where normal anxiety and reactive depression are extremely common.

The first few days after giving birth are full of intense and varied emotions. The first twenty-four hours are a period of recovery from the fatigue caused by childbirth. In general, the puerperal woman feels weak and confused, especially when the birth took place under narcosis. Emotional lability is the most characteristic pattern of the first week after childbirth: euphoria and depression alternate rapidly, and the latter can reach great intensity. Some authors believe that these symptoms are due to the biochemical changes that take place immediately after labour, such as the increased secretion of corticosteroids and the sudden drop in hormone levels.

They also involve other factors such as the frustrations and monotony of the hospitalisation period and the transition from the anxious waiting typical of the end of pregnancy to the awareness of the new reality which, alongside the satisfaction of motherhood, also means the responsibility of taking on new tasks and limiting some previous activities. It is sometimes difficult to determine the dividing line between normality and pathology in the case of post-natal depression. In any case, the intensification or permanence of depressive symptoms a few weeks after giving birth should be looked at more carefully (MALDONADO 1988).

According to Soifer (1980), in this period we see states of confusion in the parturient woman, anxiety about emptying and castration, in other words, the ambivalence between what was lost (the pregnancy) and what was acquired (the child). An important aspect is that, for the mother, the reality of the **foetus "in utero" is not the same as the reality of the** newborn baby and for many women it is difficult to make this transition, especially those with a strong infantile dependence on their mother or husband. They can easily love their child while it is still inside them and love an idealised image of the baby, but not the reality of the newborn.

The author's observations show that this occurs mainly in women who **tend to believe that their baby will be "different" (calm, crying little, sleeping at night** from the start, etc.), denying in advance the reality of a baby in the first few weeks of life, before whom they often feel frightened and confused about the responsibility of maternal care. (SOIFER, 1980, p.75).

In Maldonado's view, during pregnancy, the child is often felt to be part of the mother's body and, for this reason, the birth can be experienced as an amputation. After giving birth, the woman realises that the baby is someone else: it becomes necessary to elaborate the loss of the baby from the fantasy in order to enter into real contact (MALDONADO, 1985, p.76).

2.3 What life is like for a woman with post-natal depression

According to Winnicott (1988), during pregnancy women are pampered and surrounded by affectionate looks. But all attention is focused on her belly; it's as if at this moment she becomes "a belly". In general, her entire investment becomes centred on her baby: the preparations, the care for its health and the expectations and fantasies about what it will be like. This magical state of fulfilment is broken with the birth of the baby and all the magic of birth is transformed into the reality of a concrete baby, who doesn't always live up to all expectations.

At the same time, the woman's body is touched by the pain, by the cut, and it doesn't go back to the way it was so quickly. Reality and fantasy collide, bringing certain conflicts that are not always well absorbed by the woman. As a result, the woman may experience moments of anguish (WINNICOTT, 1988).

The puerperal woman's first anxiety is about breastfeeding, wondering if she will have enough milk or even if the baby will accept it. Staying in hospital is felt to be soothing, in the sense that it provides the puerperal woman and her child with all the assistance and care they need. The day of hospital discharge arrives and, with it, the return home. The fear of taking responsibility for the baby alone increases maternal insecurity. In addition, the special attention, celebrations and visits begin to diminish, while the obligations take on immense proportions. Anxieties about motherhood intensify once again (WINNICOTT, 1988).

The fear of not living up to the idealised mother figure is combined with the fear of not knowing how to look after the baby, creating the possibility that it will fall ill and die. The first ten days after giving birth are the worst. The confrontation with her current body is a difficult aspect to overcome, as she had become accustomed to the image of her pregnant body. Although empty, she doesn't recognise it as being the same as it was before pregnancy or at any other time in her life (WINNICOTT, 1988).

Another maternal anxiety is sharing the baby with other people, including the child's own father, because while pregnant she had an exclusive relationship with him, which was felt to be hers alone (WINNICOTT, 1988).

Many women feel disappointed in their partners because they feel they are not receiving the support and affection they expected, or because they feel indifferent towards the baby. As the woman is the source of the baby, the bond between her and the baby is gradually established
This doesn't happen with the father who, during this period, sees himself as a mere spectator, often forgetting that he also helped to bring about conception. In this way, the bond between father and baby is formed more slowly, also because at first the child is perceived as a great rival, as he mobilises all the attention and care of his partner. As a result, many fathers will feel abandoned and in need of support and comfort, as they are also anxious and fearful about the present and future and wonder if they will be able to provide for and protect the new family. Many also find it difficult to resume an active sex life for fear of hurting the woman or because they realise how tired and confused they feel with their new responsibilities, or even because they are jealous and envious of the intimate mother-baby relationship, especially when breastfeeding, when they feel excluded from the relationship (WINNICOTT, 1988).

CHAPTER 3

OCCUPATIONAL THERAPY CARE STRATEGY

According to Magalhães (2005), we can say that man has been part of different groups since birth. Men are born, grow up, develop and die as part of different social groups. They dialectically seek to establish an individual identity, but also a group identity. In fact, man is, by nature, an essentially gregarious animal.

Generally speaking, groups can be categorised in different ways, which vary according to the degree of kinship, the purpose for which they are intended, etc. We can refer to family groups, religious groups, school groups, therapeutic groups and a whole range of other social groups.

From the point of view of Occupational Therapy, the perspective of using activities with groups has been systematically employed in the USA since the 1930s. The initial focus given to work developed with groups, especially in the area of mental health, was related to socialisation objectives.

In the 60s, 70s and 80s, the use of groups as a form of treatment intensified. Numerous studies were carried out in the United States by occupational therapists such as Gail Fidler, Mosey, Schuman and others. Studies that analyse and describe groups and activities based on different approaches, such as psychodynamic, behavioural, developmental and so on.

In Brazil, it can be seen that during the 1980s and 1990s, occupational therapists widely used group therapy. It can be seen that these professionals developed therapeutic groups with a very diverse clientele in terms of age group and the problems presented. Occupational therapists have worked with groups of elderly people, psychotic patients, children with neurological problems, among others (MAGALHÃES, 2005, p.65-67).

Given the high number of women with emotional disorders after pregnancy who are diagnosed with post-natal depression or whose pathology has not been identified due to a lack of professionals and specialised care to establish such a diagnosis, the formation of a group of pregnant women with an occupational therapist during prenatal care could help to identify, prevent or alleviate future post-natal depression.

In a therapeutic group, the aim is to treat the group participants, unlike a social group. In a therapeutic group, the effective presence of the therapist is necessary for treatment to take place. It is assumed that the therapist can offer the group members the opportunity to get to know each other through their interventions and interpretations (MAGALHÃES, 2005, p.67).

In occupational therapy, considering a psychodynamic approach, an activity group can be defined as one in which the participants get together in the presence of the occupational therapist to experience things related to doing, such as: walking, painting, drawing, modelling, dancing, shopping, relaxing, playing games, sewing, etc. We can also consider that the aim of an occupational therapy activity group is treatment and all that it entails.

Another essential aspect that we must emphasise is that one of the principles that surrounds the clinical practice of the occupational therapist is related to the idea that doing has a therapeutic effect. We start from the understanding that all the elements that relate to doing - such as the choice and indication of the activity, the actual realisation of the end product, as well as the relationship that is established throughout the occupational therapy process between the therapist, the patient and the group - are of fundamental importance.

Understanding the patient as a whole, according to Benneton (1994), makes it possible to establish a situational diagnosis. This formulation seems extremely important to us, because the perspective of trying to understand the patient in their entirety (their life, family, occupational history, etc.) and, above all, understanding and diagnosing the situation and conditions (way of relating, general state, pragmatism) presented by the patient at the time of referring and selecting them for the group are of fundamental importance to the occupational therapist. (MAGALHÃES, 2005, p.68 to 71).

In a group where all the participants are pregnant women undergoing prenatal care, the occupational therapist, as the scientist of human occupation, will use the activity to carry out his therapeutic process with the aim of expressing emotions, doubts, fears, rejections, expectations, anxieties, in other words, all the feelings and questions raised by the women.

With these feelings expressed, the occupational therapist will establish the treatment plan, the material to be used, select according to demand and identify whether any of them already have symptoms characteristic of developing post-natal depression.

After diagnosing the symptoms, they will be worked on by the occupational therapist through activity, as this is understood as a stimulus, as a central element of the occupational therapeutic process, as a mediator of the therapeutic relationship, as a form of expression of the patients' inner contents.

The way in which groups are set up in an institution, specifically activity groups, is not the same. We must take into account the diversity of aspects, ranging from the profile of the clientele served, the objectives of the service and treatment, to the composition of the technical team (MAGALHÃES, 2005, p.70).

For an activity group to be set up, we understand that the role played by the occupational therapist in the preparation and planning stage of the group is of fundamental importance.

Aspects pertaining to the characteristics of the group - number of participants, referrals, selection criteria, establishment of the therapeutic contract, preparation of the environment and materials - must be carefully assessed by the occupational therapist who will be coordinating the activity group.

We may come across activity groups with 16 participants and others with three. Our clinical experience has shown us that considering the conditions in which the participants find themselves can be an indicator that contributes to determining the most appropriate number for setting up the group. In general, groups made up of between five and eight participants have proved to be viable, especially in the area of mental health (MAGALHÃES, 2005, p.70 to 72).

In the case of the group formed by women in prenatal care, the structure of the group will be homogeneous and open, i.e. a homogeneous group is one in which the participants have common disorders (women who are going through the period of pregnancy and who may have common feelings, fears and doubts) and an open group is one in which the participants can be replaced by other members when they drop out. As we are talking about a group of patients who are in different periods of pregnancy, at any moment a birth may occur and this woman can be replaced by another who is starting prenatal care, as the treatment plan will be established by the occupational therapist according to the demand presented by the patient. (MAGALHÃES 2005, p.70 to 75).

With the birth of these babies, the therapist should monitor these women's puerperium. Seven days after the birth, the occupational therapist can apply the Edinburgh scale, which identifies symptoms and establishes a diagnosis of post-natal depression. Once the pathology has been diagnosed, the therapist can work individually with each puerperal woman. If no symptoms appear initially, the therapist will be able to accompany her until the fourth month after the birth of the baby, which is approximately the period when depression can appear.

CHAPTER 4

METHODOLOGY

This research was carried out at the Integrated Coordination Centre for Women's, Children's and Adolescents' Health in the city of Carmo, Rio de Janeiro. A data survey was carried out at this institution to find out what kind of care these women receive during the prenatal period, what care they receive during the puerperium, whether there is any therapeutic follow-up and what programme is offered there by the government.

An adapted semi-structured instrument, the Edinburgh Scale, was also applied to women who had already been diagnosed with post-natal depression, in a group of 120 women treated by the institution.

Among the existing self-assessment scales, the Edinburgh Postnatal Depression Scale (EPDS) is the most widely used for screening depressive symptoms that manifest after childbirth, and has been translated into several languages, with validation studies in most countries (SANTOS MFS, 1995).

The Edinburgh Rating Scale (EPDS) consists of a self-report instrument made up of 10 statements, the options for which are scored (0 to 3) according to the presence or intensity of the symptom. Its items cover psychological symptoms such as depressed mood (feelings of sadness, self-worth and guilt, ideas of death or suicide), loss of pleasure in activities previously considered enjoyable, fatigue, decreased ability to think, concentrate or make decisions, as well as physiological symptoms (insomnia or hypersomnia) and behavioural changes (crying spells).The sum of the points makes a score of 30, with a value equal to or greater than 12 being considered depressive symptomatology, as defined in the validation of the scale in a Brazilian sample.(SANTOS MFS,1995).

With the appropriate adaptation of the Edinburgh Scale, the instrument is called semi-structured, where the interviewee has the opportunity to discuss the proposed topic, without answers or conditions set by the interviewer. The script is much more flexible, meaning that the interview technique becomes a more spontaneous, informal conversation. The aim is to find out how important therapeutic care is for women during the antenatal period and whether there is a demand for it.

Before starting to apply the research instrument, the Municipal Health Department of the city of Carmo RJ was given a consent form explaining the objectives of the research and obtaining permission for the full access required during the research. A consent and clarification form was also given to the coordinator responsible for the institution.

In the course of preparing the research, a very thorough study was made of postnatal depression, its causes, symptoms, risk factors, the intervention of occupational therapy, the importance of prenatal care and therapeutic care in the puerperium, the emergence of women in society and the importance of motherhood since the beginning.

For this research, we studied texts, bibliographical reviews, research articles, research theses, experience reports and websites related to motherhood/pregnancy/pregnancy.

CHAPTER 5

DATA ANALYSIS AND DISCUSSION

During a survey carried out at the Women's Health Centre of the Carmo City Hall in Rio de Janeiro between April 2009 and May 2009, we found that the centre currently provides antenatal care to 120 pregnant women. These pregnant women are seen by obstetricians, gynaecologists, nurses and nutritionists. These women do not receive any therapeutic care during their prenatal care.

With the birth of the child, care is provided at another integrated institution and during this time the woman answers a clinical gynaecological questionnaire. The newborn undergoes medical treatment, examinations, a baby's foot test, vaccinations, etc.

The Rio de Janeiro state government's PAISMCA programme was set up in 1998 and the Integrated Coordination Centre for Women's, Children's and Adolescents' Health in 2005, and so far only one case of post-natal depression has been diagnosed. The psychological condition was only recognised because the woman already had psychiatric disorders and was referred to the institution for assistance.

This is one of the factors that proves the importance of the multi-professional team. If, during the prenatal period, these women were not only attended to by the primary care team, but were also offered the services of an Occupational Therapist, possible symptoms of future post-natal depression could appear and these could be worked on therapeutically in Occupational Therapy to reverse them or even to try to prevent or alleviate possible post-natal depression.

In addition to PAISMCA, the institution has other government programmes, including SISPRENATAL. Currently, 9 professionals are working there: 2 gynaecologists and obstetricians, 2 nurses, 1 coordinator of the Women's, Adolescents' and Children's Health C.C.I. (head of department), 2 nursing assistants, 1 administrative assistant and 1 nutritionist.

In the future, the institution plans to offer these mothers care during the puerperium. The following is the full report of the opinion of nurse M. F. M., coordinator of PAISMCA at this institution, on occupational therapy during the prenatal and puerperium periods.

TABLE 4: Report from the Head of Nursing at the Institution

Fragment of the speech by nurse M.F.M., coordinator of PAISMCA.
The multi-professional team is of paramount importance at any level of health care. When it comes to women's health, this assistance becomes fundamental. Although a multi-professional team already works here, it needs to be expanded and improved in order to better meet the needs not only of pregnant women, but also adolescents, women of childbearing age and postpartum women.

Source: Field research 2009.

Based on nurse Maria F. M's speech, we believe that the presence of an Occupational Therapist in the team is relevant so that the emotional aspect of these mothers can be therapeutically monitored. If any mothers show symptoms of post-natal depression, they will be assessed and diagnosed. Once post-natal depression has been diagnosed, these mothers will continue to receive care from the Occupational Therapist and will be referred to other specialised professionals.

Most of the time, pregnant women in Brazil are seen by public institutions as if they were just a belly and forget about their emotional side. As a result, many suffer from post-natal depression, but it is not treated correctly because it is not diagnosed due to a lack of professionals to recognise and treat the case.

Given that cases of post-natal depression are not diagnosed, many women have the condition and go through enormous suffering without knowing what they are really suffering from, and as a result there are no records of women who have the condition. We therefore carried out a field study in which we found 10 cases of women diagnosed with post-natal depression.

The data presented below was collected by applying an adapted semi-structured instrument, the Edinburgh Scale, to women with diagnosed postnatal depression.

The following graph refers to the women who answered the questionnaire and those who refused to have post-natal depression for some reason.

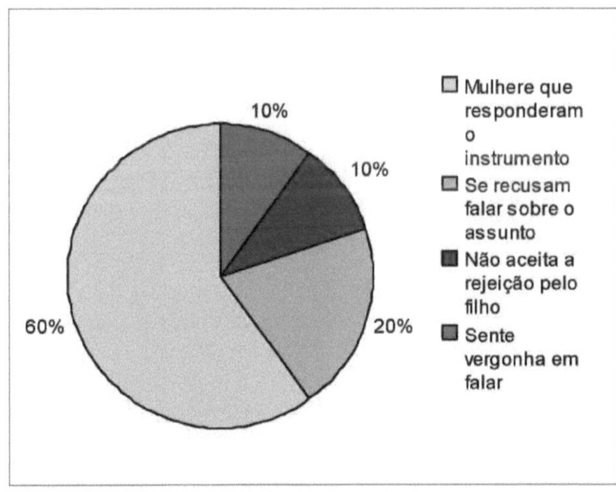

FIGURA 1: **Instrument**
Source: Field research 2009

In the graph above, only 60 per cent of the women selected agreed to answer the questionnaire and talk about it. 20 per cent refused to talk about it for some reason, 10 per cent didn't accept the rejection they were currently feeling from their child and the remaining 10 per cent felt ashamed of showing post-natal depression.

In order to construct the following graphs, the postpartum women answered the following questions that make up the Edinburgh Scale.

TABLE 5: Edinburgh Scale

Have you been able to laugh and find things funny lately?
Do you feel pleasure when you think about what's going on in your day-to-day life?
Have you been blaming yourself unnecessarily when things go wrong?
Have you been feeling anxious or worried for no good reason?
Have you been feeling scared or panicked?
Have you been feeling overwhelmed by the tasks and events of your day-to-day life?
Have you been feeling so unhappy that you can't sleep?
Do you feel sad or devastated?
Have you been feeling so unhappy that you've been crying?
Has the thought of harming yourself ever crossed your mind?

The results for these questions are represented by the following graphs respectively:

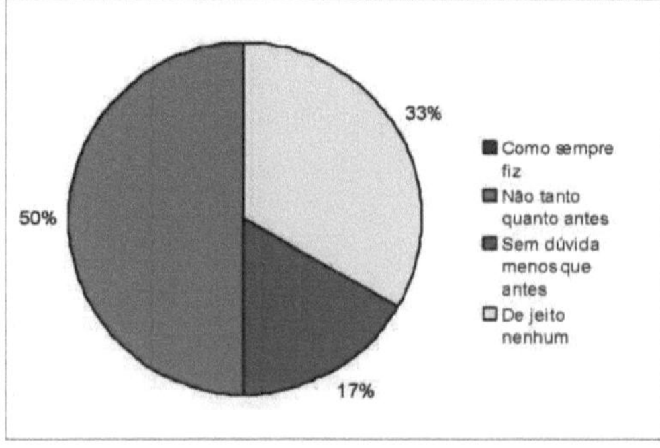

Source: Field research 2009.

In the graph above, 50 per cent of the women said that they don't smile as much as they did before they had children, but they still smile. 33% said that they no longer smile at all and 17% said that they do smile, but definitely less than before.

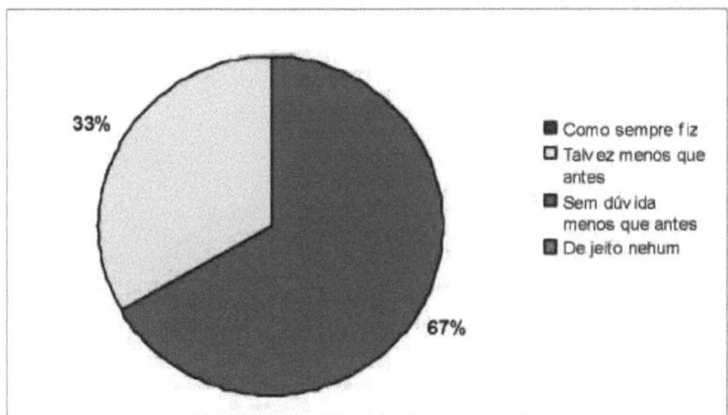

FIGURA 3:   **Activities of daily living**

Source: Field research 2009.

In the graph above, 33 per cent of the women said that they felt less pleasure in activities of daily living than before having children and the other 67 per cent reported that they definitely felt less pleasure than before.

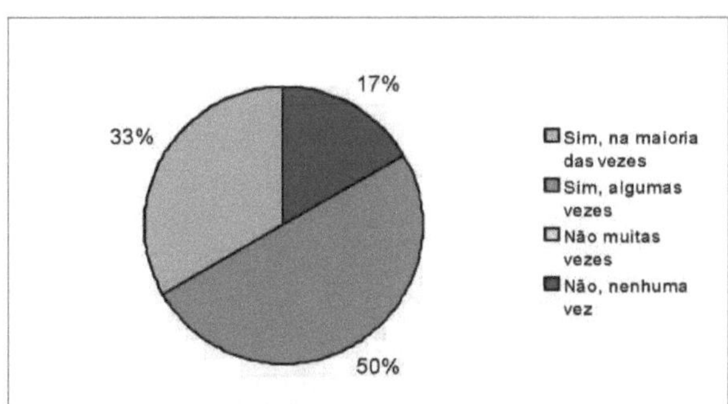

FIGURA 4:   **Feelings of guilt**
Source: Field research 2009

In the graph above, 50 per cent of women say they feel guilty unnecessarily when something goes wrong. 33% say they feel guilty most of the time and 17% say they don't feel guilty at all.

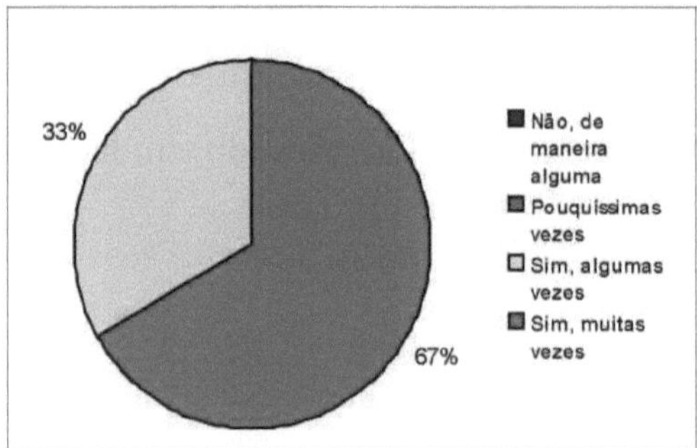

FIGURA 5: **Anxiety and Worry**
Source: Field research 2009.

In the graph above, 67 per cent of the women reported that they often feel worried and anxious for no good reason and 33 per cent said that they experience these feelings sometimes.

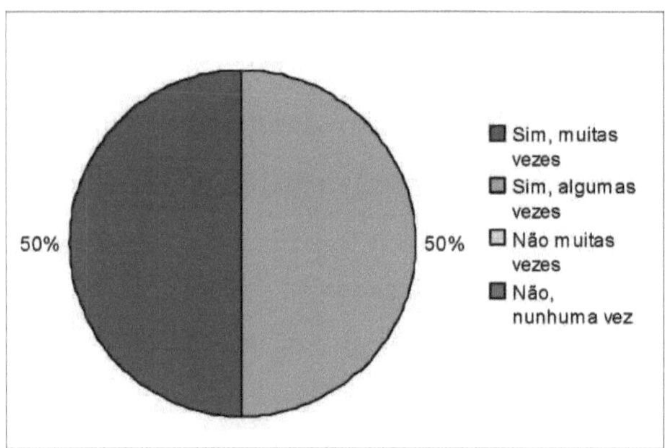

FIGURA 6: **Feeling of panic**

Source: Field research 2009.

In the graph above, 50 per cent of the women said they felt panicked often for no reason and 50 per cent said they felt it sometimes. In other words, the feeling of panic is somehow present in the lives of all these women.

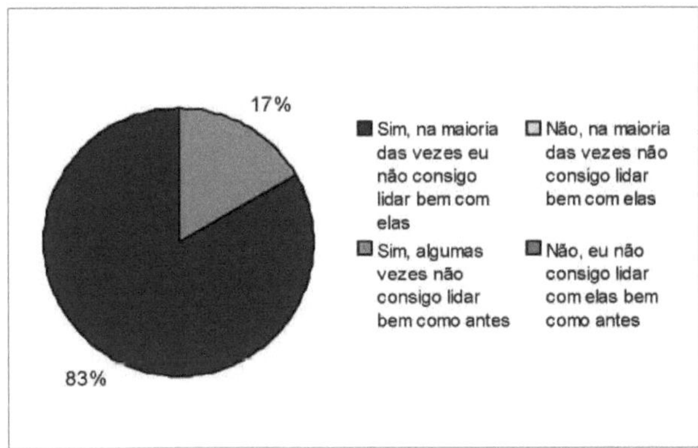

FIGURA 7: **She feels exhausted**
Source: Field research 2009

In the graph above, 83 per cent of the women reported that most of the time they were unable to carry out their activities of daily living because they felt exhausted and 17 per cent said that sometimes they were able to carry out their activities, but not as well as before.

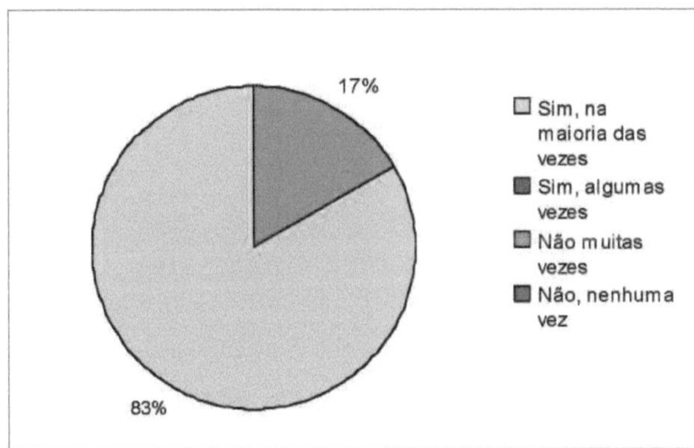

FIGURA 8: **Feeling of unhappiness**
Source: Field research 2009

In the graph above, 83 per cent of women reported that they were so unhappy that they could no longer sleep and 17 per cent said that it wasn't often that their unhappiness got in the way of sleeping.

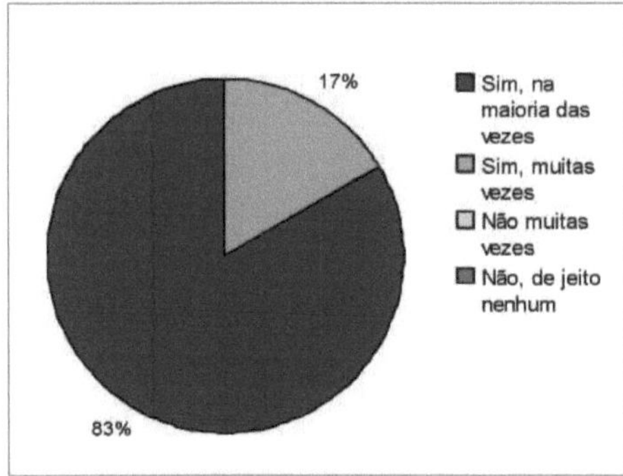

FIGURA 9: **Feeling of sadness**
Source: Field research 2009

In the graph above, 83 per cent of the women reported that most of the time they felt sad or devastated and 17 per cent said that they felt this way a lot. This graph shows that the feeling of sadness is constantly present in these women's lives.

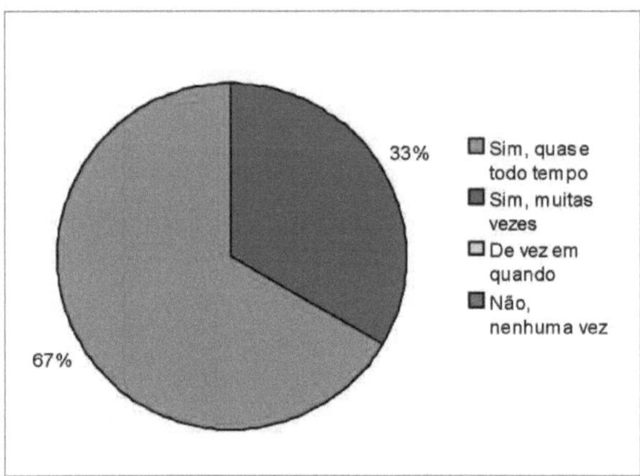

FIGURA 10: **He finds himself crying**
Source: Field research 2009.

In the graph above, 67 per cent of the women said they were so sad that they cried and 33 per cent said they cried many times a day. Crying is a constant in these women's lives, several times a day.

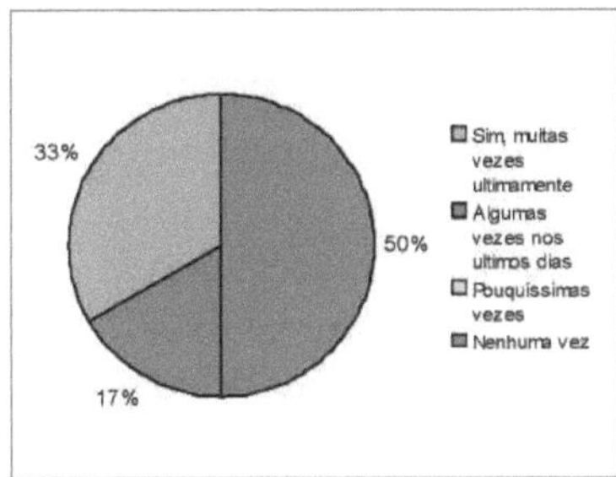

FIGURA 11: **Suicidal thoughts**
Source: Field research 2009.

This graph represents 50 per cent of the women who said they had never thought about harming themselves, 33 per cent said they had often thought about it recently and 17 per cent had thought about it a few times in recent days.

The following are excerpts from reports that have been transcribed in full, without correcting the cultured norm, of these women's opinions on the implementation of occupational therapy in prenatal care.

TABLE 6: Interviewees' accounts

What do you think of a preventive occupational therapy programme to support pregnant women as a complementary part of prenatal care? Do you think it would prevent possible post-natal depression?
I think it would have helped a lot. In my case, for example, I realise that if I'd had this antenatal care, I wouldn't have had *the* depression. It was an unplanned pregnancy, much less a wanted one, and I was having problems with my husband. I think therapy would have helped me resolve these conflicts in my head. For me, it would have prevented it.
I think it would help a lot. In my case, I had mixed feelings and needed help to understand myself. I was completely lost and agonised.
I think it would help. But each case is different. In mine, for example, it would help, but at the moment I'd think it was unimportant because I apparently didn't feel anything during my pregnancy. It would help a lot because when you get pregnant you think everything is a fairytale, as if the baby that's about to arrive is a "doll", but when it's born, you realise that everything is completely different, your life changes 100%,

I thought I was prepared, but I wasn't. I'm not.
No doubt about it. I think pregnant women should start receiving occupational therapy from the moment they find out they're pregnant.
Yes, it would. We become very sensitive during pregnancy. I think this therapy would even help the baby, since *the* child feels everything that's going on through its mother. It would be great, there are so many things a therapist could work on in a woman's emotional life. What's more, I think the fathers could be counselled too, they need to know about the enormous changes that are happening to the woman, so that they can understand and help her.
I think it's great. I was going through a huge disappointment, I'd split up and only with counselling could I have felt better. Of course it would prevent it, at least for me. I was needy, confused and had a lot of fears about carrying on with my pregnancy. I was even afraid that I wouldn't be able to look after and educate my son.

Source: Field research 2009.

CHAPTER 6

CONCLUSION

This study shows that postnatal depression is a common psychological condition among women. It is a severe and acute clinical condition that can begin in the first week after giving birth. Inability to care, overzealousness and lack of interest in the baby are just three of the symptoms of postnatal depression that affect not only the mother but also the child.

There are three types of clinical depression in the postnatal period: Blues (mild disorder), Postpartum Depression and Postpartum Psychosis (severe disorder). Most of the time this condition is not diagnosed and treated correctly due to the lack of specialised professionals working in this area.

The government of the state of Rio de Janeiro offers various programmes for women's health care through the SUS (single health system), but without a complete multi-professional team, these puerperal women are not seen as a whole and most of the time, pregnant women are treated as if they were just a belly and their emotional state is forgotten. As a result, post-natal depression is not very reliable and is not always treated.

Pregnancy and childbirth are stressful events that can in themselves contribute to the onset of depression. During this period, women are more sensitive and often confused. It is because of these conditions that therapeutic care during the antenatal period plays a major role in preventing postnatal depression.

We can also conclude that the aim of a group of activities in Occupational Therapy is treatment and all that it entails and the principles surrounding clinical practice is that doing has a therapeutic effect.

Occupational therapy can help prevent or alleviate future post-natal depression in cases that have already been diagnosed, since occupational therapy can improve the quality of life of these women through activity.

CHAPTER 7

BIBLIOGRAPHICAL REFERENCES

ARGERAMI. Valdemar Augusto. **Hospital Psychology:** Theory and Practice. São Paulo: Editora Thomson pioneira, 2006.

BURROUGHS, Arlene. **An introduction to**: Maternal Nursing. 6 ed. Porto Alegre: Editora Artes Médicas, 1995.

CAMARGO, R. et al. **Anatomy for movement**. Translator: Sophie Guernet. São Paulo: Manole, 1991.

CURY, Augusto. **Mary:** the greatest educator in history. Editora Planeta do Brasil. São Paulo, 2007.

GARDNER, E. **Anatomy:** Regional study of the human body. Translator: Rogério Benevento. 4. ed. Rio de Janeiro: Guanabara Koogan, 1988.

KAPLAN, Harold I Kaplan, Benjamin J. Sadock, Jack[a] Grebb. Porto Alegre: Artmed publishing house, 8[a] ed, 2007.

MAGALHÃES, Lílian Vieira. et.al: **Occupational Therapy:** Theory and Practice. 3aed.Papirus. Campinas, 2005.

MALDONADO, Maria Tereza. **Psychology of pregnancy**. Petrópolis: Editora Vozes, 7th edition, 1985.

MOREIRA, Patrícia Rose Teixeira: **Art Therapy**: Start where you are by building your own image. Maceió 2006/2007.

MINISTRY OF HEALTH. Technical Manual: prenatal and puerperium care, qualified and humanised. Brasilia, 2006.

PALASTANA, N. et al. **Anatomy and human movement**: structure and function. Translation: Nelson Gomes de Oliveira. São Paulo: Manole, 2000.

PSYCHIATRY, Brazilian Association of. Available at: <http://www.abpbrasil.org.br/ Accessed November 2008

SABOTTA, Johannes. Sabotta **Atlas of Human Anatomy**. Rio de Janeiro: Guanabara, Koogan, 2000.

SANTOS MFS. **Postpartum depression:** Validation of the Edinburgh Scale in Brazilian puerperal women [thesis]: Brasília: University of Brasília; 1995.

SOIFER, Raquel. **Psychology of Pregnancy, Childbirth and the Puerperium.** Porto Alegre: Editora: Artes Médicas, 1980.

WINNICOTT, D.W. **Babies and their Mothers**. Psychology and Pedagogy Collection. São Paulo: Martins Fontes, 1988.

ZIMERMAN DE. **Technical fundamentals.** In Zimerman DE; Osório LC. (et al) How we work with groups. Porto Alegre: Artes Médicas.

CHAPTER 8

ANNEXES

MAIN SYMPTOMS
Depressed mood, where the intensity and depth of the pain becomes so unbearable that it often generates the desire for death as a solution. This feeling lasts long enough to seem like a permanent state.
A feeling of sadness that occurs spontaneously without being associated with any relevant fact. This feeling resists being changed even in the face of clear observation, logical reasoning or external appeal and encouragement.
Loss of interest even in things that were once special and interesting (anhedonia). Depressed people often neglect and abandon most of the things they once valued in life, such as family and profession. They realise their sadness and affective abandonment, but they still can't react, keeping their lives within a day-to-day routine without expectations or energy.
Difficulty concentrating, low self-esteem, loss of self-confidence, hopelessness, self-depreciation, self-reproach, feelings of worthlessness and incapacity even for things that are recognised as capable.
Loss of life expectancy, suicidal thoughts and the carrying out of "small suicidal acts and rehearsals," such as exposing oneself to risky situations and disregarding dangers.
Increased use and abuse of substances, especially cocaine, alcohol and medication.
Chronic pain or other persistent bodily symptoms that have no obvious clinical justification - among the most recurrent clinical complaints are: constant colds, back pain, anorgasmia (absence of orgasm), tremors; changes in blood pressure, impotence, skin expressions; loss of muscle strength, others.
Presence of facial masks (facial inexpressiveness)
Poor speech and expression

Inability to move in the direction of the necessary and even the essential, such as bathing, eating, working, etc...
Motor agitation or, on the other hand, a certain motor and intellectual retardation that can also oscillate between them (bipolarity). Agitation is usually accompanied by anxiety, irritability and aggression, in contrast to a certain slowness in body movements.
Severe episodes of depression include some psychotic symptoms. The most common are hallucinations (hearing or seeing) and delusions (magical thoughts that hold opinions in a rigid and unprovable way without, however, being based on or explained by any concept of logic).
Other common symptoms are melancholy, subtle or profound disturbances in eating and sleeping, decreased sex drive and unspecified bodily discomfort.

Source: Programme to combat depression.

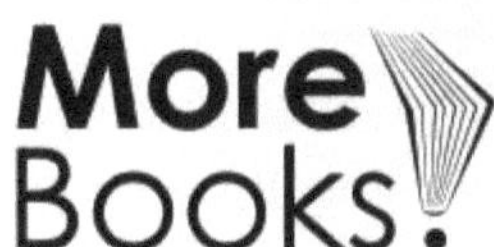

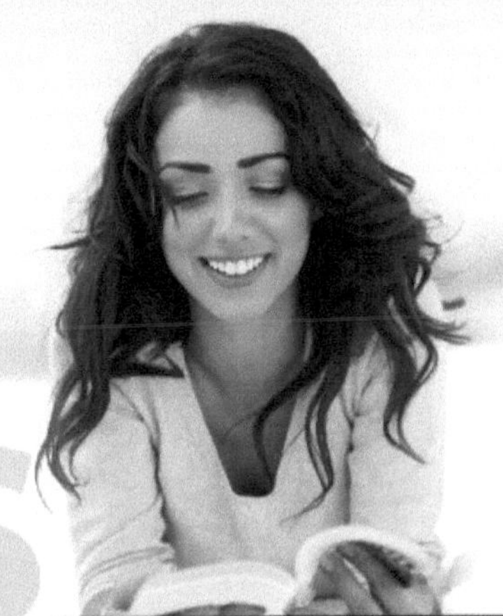

Buy your books fast and straightforward online - at one of world's fastest growing online book stores! Environmentally sound due to Print-on-Demand technologies.

Buy your books online at
www.morebooks.shop

Kaufen Sie Ihre Bücher schnell und unkompliziert online – auf einer der am schnellsten wachsenden Buchhandelsplattformen weltweit! Dank Print-On-Demand umwelt- und ressourcenschonend produziert.

Bücher schneller online kaufen
www.morebooks.shop

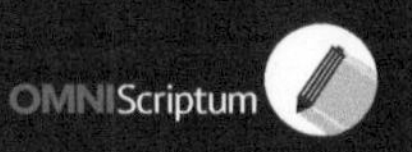

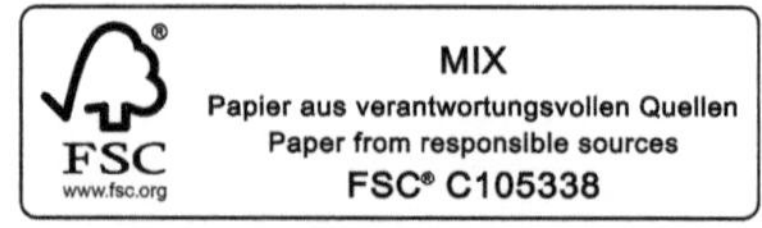

Printed by Books on Demand GmbH, Norderstedt / Germany